WHAT LONGEVITY MEANS

The Secret of Living Well and Longer

By

Kurt Banks

Table of Contents

Introduction

What Does Longevity Mean

Longevity is the ability to live a long and healthy life.

It is a topic that has fascinated humans for centuries, as people have always been intrigued by the possibility of living longer and healthier lives.

Longevity has different meanings to different people, depending on their culture, beliefs, and personal experiences.

To many, longevity means the ability to live a full and healthy life, free from illness and disease. It involves being able to maintain physical, mental, and emotional well-being throughout one's lifespan, as well as having a strong social support system to provide companionship and assistance when needed.

Others may see longevity as a way to achieve their life goals and aspirations.

They may view a long life as an opportunity to make a positive impact on the world and leave a lasting legacy for future generations.

This could involve pursuing a fulfilling career, contributing to their community, or creating works of art or literature that will inspire others.

In some cultures, longevity is highly valued and celebrated as a sign of wisdom, respect, and honour.

In many Asian cultures, for example, there is a long tradition of respecting and honouring the elderly, who are seen as repositories of knowledge and wisdom.

Longevity holds great significance for humans, as it represents our innate desire to live long, fulfilling lives and leave a positive mark on the world.

While achieving longevity may require making certain lifestyle choices and adopting healthy habits, it is ultimately a reflection of our ability to adapt and thrive in the face of life's challenges and uncertainties.

Chapter 1

Longevity Vs. Life Expectancy

Understanding life expectancy is a critical piece of the puzzle in the pursuit of longevity.

Life expectancy, generally defined as the average number of years a person is expected to live, is an important indicator that represents a population's overall health and well-being.

The Historical Context

Over the course of human history, life expectancy has increased dramatically.

Our forefathers encountered several problems that drastically shortened life expectancy in ancient times.

Infectious diseases, high infant mortality rates, a lack of medical knowledge, and poor living conditions all contributed to short lifespans. In reality, in the pre-modern age, it was typical for people to die in their 30s or 40s.

This landscape was revolutionized by the introduction of modern medicine, greater sanitation, and developments in public health initiatives. Life expectancy increased dramatically in the twentieth century, with many countries experiencing a doubling or more of the average lifespan. These increases were mostly credited to technological advancements such as antibiotics, vaccinations, and improved healthcare infrastructure.

Today's Life Expectancy

Today, life expectancy varies greatly around the globe. Because of better healthcare, nutrition, and living conditions, high-income countries have longer life expectancies than low-income countries.

However, differences can occur even within the same country. The global average life expectancy was roughly 73 years as of the end of 2021.

It is crucial to remember, however, that this figure may fluctuate over time as civilizations and healthcare systems adapt.

Chapter 2

How Longevity Pays

Longevity, or the ability to live a longer life, has a plethora of possible advantages.

While the pursuit of a longer lifespan has long been a goal for humans, it is critical to understand that living longer should ideally be accompanied by living better—maintaining good health and well-being as we age.

Here are some of the advantages of living a long life:

Extended Quality Time with Loved Ones:

Spending extra time with family and friends is one of the most treasured benefits of longevity. Longer life gives more opportunities to create treasured memories with loved ones, to witness the growth of children and grandkids, and to reinforce the links that bind families together.

Greater Personal Fulfilment:

Living a longer life allows one more time to pursue personal objectives and interests. Longevity allows people to explore and accomplish their aspirations, whether they are touring the world, starting a new career, or taking up a hobby.

Wisdom Accumulation:

Wisdom generally comes with age. Longer lives allow for more opportunities to learn from life events, which can lead to more wisdom and a better understanding of oneself and the world.

Contribution to Society:

Many older people continue to contribute significantly to society through voluntary work, mentoring, or even second professions.

Their life experiences and knowledge are extremely beneficial to their communities.

Economic Benefits:

Living longer can allow you to acquire more wealth and assets, resulting in greater financial security in retirement. This can also benefit the general economy because older people continue to engage in economic activity.

Increased Innovation:

Living longer can translate into more production. This longer working life can stimulate creativity since older people offer their experience and expertise to a variety of disciplines, contributing to technological, scientific, and cultural developments.

Social Connection and Networks:

Longevity generally allows for the development of deeper social relationships and networks. Strong social networks can offer emotional support, alleviate loneliness, and increase general well-being.

Positive Effects on Communities:

Longer lives can lead to more stable communities since older people typically contribute to community cohesion and social capital through their involvement in local organizations and activities.

Greater Time for Personal Development:

Longevity provides the gift of time for personal development and self-improvement. Individuals can pursue new hobbies, learn new talents, and continue to grow personally throughout their lives.

Transcending Generational Boundaries:

As people live longer lives, they are able to overcome generational barriers, increasing intergenerational understanding, cooperation, and empathy.

Legacy and Impact:

Living longer enables people to leave a greater legacy and impact on future generations. They have the ability to pass down knowledge, values, and experiences that will impact others.

Adaptation to Changing Times:

Living longer requires adapting to changing conditions and embracing lifelong learning. This adaptation has the potential to lead to a more fulfilling and resilient existence.

Chapter 3

Factors That Influence Longevity

Longevity is influenced by multiple factors, including genetics, lifestyle choices, access to healthcare, environmental, social, mental factors et. al.

While there is no single formula for living a long and healthy life, understanding these factors can help individuals make informed decisions about their health and well-being.

i. Genetics

Genetics account for about 25% of human lifespan variation, with certain mutations linked to premature ageing and diseases like cancer.

Some genetic variations, such as those affecting DNA repair mechanisms, have been associated with longer lifespans. For example, certain FOXO3A gene variants increase the chance of living to 100 or older.

However, genetics only account for a portion of lifespan variation, with lifestyle and environmental factors playing a greater role.

Overall, genetics and lifestyle factors play a crucial role in determining an individual's lifespan.

ii. Lifestyle Choices

Lifestyle choices, including diet, exercise, and smoking habits, significantly impact longevity.

Regular physical activity, maintaining a healthy weight, and avoiding smoking and excessive alcohol consumption are linked to longer and healthier lives.

Lifestyle factors such as a healthy diet, weight management, avoiding harmful substances like tobacco and excessive alcohol consumption, and stress management are also strongly associated with longevity.

Diet: A diet rich in whole foods, including fruits, vegetables, whole grains, and lean proteins, is linked to a lower risk of chronic diseases and a longer lifespan.

Conversely, diets high in processed foods, saturated fats, and added sugars increase the risk of obesity, heart disease, and other chronic conditions which can reduce lifespan.

Exercise: Regular physical activity can reduce the risk of chronic diseases, improve cardiovascular health, and enhance overall well-being.

Studies show that moderate-intensity exercise, like brisk walking or cycling, lowers the risk of premature death compared to inactivity. To achieve this, aim for at least 30 minutes of moderate-intensity exercise on most days of the week, such as walking, jogging, cycling, or swimming.

Get Adequate Sleep: Sleep plays an important role in overall health, and getting enough restful sleep is essential for maintaining good health and preventing chronic diseases. Aim for 7-8 hours of sleep per night and establish a consistent sleep schedule.

Maintain a Healthy Weight: Being overweight or obese can increase the risk of chronic diseases such as heart disease, diabetes, and cancer, and reduce lifespan. Maintaining a healthy weight through regular exercise and a balanced diet can help prevent these conditions.

Smoking: Smoking is a significant risk factor for various chronic diseases, including lung cancer, heart disease, and stroke.

Quitting smoking is one of the most effective ways to improve health outcomes and increase longevity.

Avoid Harmful Substances: Avoiding harmful substances such as tobacco, excessive alcohol consumption, and illicit drugs can help prevent a range of chronic diseases and increase lifespan.

iii. Environmental Factors

Environmental factors like air pollution, toxins, and access to clean water and nutritious food significantly impact longevity.

High levels of air pollution increase the risk of respiratory and cardiovascular diseases.

Access to clean water and nutritious food is crucial for maintaining good health and preventing disease.

Living in areas with better environmental quality generally leads to longer lifespans than those in poorer conditions.

iv. Access to Healthcare

Healthcare access is a crucial factor in influencing longevity.

Access to effective treatments and medications is essential for managing chronic conditions and reducing complications.

Quality healthcare, including preventive care, early disease detection, and treatment, is a strong predictor of longevity.

Individuals with regular check-ups, screenings, and vaccinations generally live longer and have better health outcomes.

v. Social Factors

Social factors like social support, education, and income level can significantly impact longevity.

Studies show that individuals with strong social connections and support systems have better health outcomes and longer lifespans. Social support helps buffer against stress's negative effects and promotes healthy behaviours, leading to longer lifespans. Therefore, social support is crucial for overall health and longevity.

Stay Socially Connected: Social support and social connections have been linked to improved health outcomes and increased lifespan. Maintaining close relationships with family and friends, volunteering, or joining social clubs can help improve social connections and overall well-being.

Education: Education is a strong predictor of longevity, with individuals who have completed more education generally living longer than those with less education. This may be due to the fact that education is associated with higher income, better healthcare access, and healthier lifestyle choices.

vi. Mental Factors

Stress and Resilience

Chronic stress can lead to health issues like high blood pressure, heart disease, and depression.

However, healthy stress management and resilience can improve overall health and longevity.

Techniques like meditation, yoga, and deep breathing exercises can help reduce stress and promote relaxation, while also increasing the risk of chronic diseases like heart disease and depression.

Maintain a Positive Attitude: A positive outlook on life can reduce stress, improve mental health, and promote overall well-being. It involves practising gratitude, engaging in joy-inducing activities, and focusing on positive experiences.

A positive attitude is linked to improved health outcomes and increased lifespan, as individuals with a sense of purpose and meaning live longer and have better mental and physical health.

Stay Mentally Engaged: Engaging in mentally stimulating activities such as reading, puzzles, and learning new skills can help improve cognitive function and reduce the risk of cognitive decline later in life.

Cognitive Function: Cognitive function, including memory and attention, has also been linked to longevity.

Individuals who maintain good cognitive function and engage in mentally stimulating activities such as reading, and puzzles generally have a lower risk of cognitive decline and may live longer.

Chapter 4

What are Longevity Supplements

Supplements have received a lot of attention as potential tools for improving longevity and overall health.

While some supplements can help with specific aspects of health, it's important to approach them with a balanced perspective and a critical eye.

In this section, we will look at the role of supplements in extending one's life, addressing both their potential benefits and the need for caution.

Supplemental Information

Supplements are products that are intended to supply essential nutrients, vitamins, minerals, amino acids, or other bioactive compounds that may be lacking in a person's diet.

They are available in a variety of forms, including pills, capsules, powders, and liquids. The goal of using supplements is to fill nutritional gaps and improve health.

The Potential Advantages of Supplements:

Supplements may provide below potential benefits for longevity and overall health:

Nutrient Deficiency Correction: For people who are deficient in certain nutrients, supplements can help restore their health. Vitamin D supplements, for example, can help combat deficiencies that are common in areas with limited sun exposure.

Supporting Specific Health Conditions: Certain supplements, such as omega-3 fatty acids for heart health or calcium and vitamin D for bone health, have shown positive effects in supporting specific health conditions, which can lead to a longer, healthier life.

Antioxidant Protection: Antioxidants such as resveratrol, as well as vitamins C and E, are thought to help combat oxidative stress and inflammation, which are linked to ageing and age-related diseases.

Cognitive Health: Omega-3 fatty acids, ginkgo biloba, and curcumin have been studied for their ability to support cognitive function and lower the risk of neurodegenerative diseases.

Bone Health: Calcium, vitamin D, and magnesium supplements can help older people maintain strong bones and reduce their risk of osteoporosis.

The Importance of Caution

While supplements can be beneficial, they must be used with caution and with the following factors in mind:

A Balanced Diet is Key: A well-balanced diet is essential. Supplements should not be used as a replacement for a well-balanced diet. Whole foods are generally the preferred way to meet nutritional needs because they provide a broader spectrum of nutrients and other bioactive compounds.

Potential for Harm: High doses of certain supplements can be harmful, even toxic. Excessive vitamin or mineral consumption can have negative consequences, including organ damage.

Lack of Regulation: The supplement industry is not as strictly regulated as the pharmaceutical industry. As a result, the quality, safety, and efficacy of supplements can vary greatly from one product to the next.

Individual Differences: What works for one person may not work for another. Individual genetics, health conditions, and lifestyle choices can all have an impact on how supplements are metabolized and their overall health impact.

Interactions with Medications: Some supplements can interact with prescription medications, potentially causing negative side effects.

Before adding supplements to your regimen, always consult a healthcare professional.

Supplements can help with longevity and overall health, but they should be viewed as a supplement to a healthy diet and lifestyle, rather than a panacea.

Before beginning any supplement regimen, speak with a healthcare provider or registered dietitian who can assess your specific nutritional needs and potential deficiencies.

Chapter 5

What are Longevity Drugs

Pharmaceutical drugs have significantly increased human life expectancy by treating and managing a variety of medical conditions.

While drugs have undoubtedly contributed to longevity, it is critical to comprehend their role in terms of both improving health and mitigating the risks associated with their use.

In this section, we will look at the various roles that pharmaceuticals play in extending one's life.

The Benefits of Pharmaceutical Drugs in Longevity

Treatment of Chronic Diseases: Many pharmaceutical drugs are required for the management of chronic conditions such as hypertension, diabetes, and heart disease. Controlling these conditions effectively can lead to a longer and healthier life.

Preventive Medications: Preventive medications, such as statins for cholesterol management or aspirin for cardiovascular health, are used to reduce the risk of life-threatening events such as heart attacks and strokes.

Antibiotics and Vaccines: Antibiotics and vaccines have been critical in reducing infectious disease mortality. Vaccination programs, in particular, have saved countless lives by preventing potentially fatal diseases.

Cancer Therapies: Advances in cancer treatments, such as chemotherapy, targeted therapies, and immunotherapies, have increased survival rates for many types of cancer, contributing to longer life.

Pain Management: Pain-relieving medications, particularly those used to treat conditions such as osteoarthritis and chronic pain, can significantly improve an individual's quality of life as they age.

Mental Health Medications: Pharmaceuticals used to treat mental health conditions such as depression, anxiety, and schizophrenia can help people live more fulfilling lives by effectively managing their symptoms.

Chapter 6

Challenges of Longevity

The Complexities and Risks of Pharmaceuticals in Achieving Longevity.

While pharmaceuticals have numerous advantages, they also have some complexities and risks.

Side Effects: Many drugs can cause side effects, some of which can be severe.

In healthcare, balancing the benefits of a medication with its potential side effects is critical.

Polypharmacy: As people age and develop multiple health conditions, they may be prescribed multiple medications, resulting in polypharmacy.

Managing multiple medications can be difficult, and it raises the risk of drug interactions and side effects.

Dependency and Tolerance: Certain drugs, particularly pain relievers and medications used to treat mental health conditions, can cause dependency and tolerance, making long-term use difficult.

Overuse and Inappropriate Use: In some cases, pharmaceuticals are overused or prescribed incorrectly, which can result in negative health outcomes. This is especially true in the context of antibiotics and opioids.

Cost and Accessibility: The cost of pharmaceutical drugs, as well as their availability to all segments of the population, can be a barrier to obtaining necessary medications, potentially affecting longevity.

Resistance: Antibiotic overuse and misuse have resulted in antibiotic resistance, a global health concern that can make treating infections more difficult and reduce the effectiveness of these drugs.

A Balanced Approach

A balanced approach is required to reap the benefits of pharmaceuticals for longevity while minimizing the risks associated with them:

Individualized Care: Healthcare should be tailored to the unique health needs of each individual, considering their medical history, genetics, and lifestyle factors.

This can aid in the optimization of drug therapy and the reduction of the risk of adverse effects.

Regular Monitoring: Regular medical check-ups and medication monitoring can help identify and address potential issues such as drug interactions, side effects, and the need for treatment adjustments.

Lifestyle Factors: A healthy lifestyle, which includes a balanced diet, regular exercise, stress management, and the avoidance of harmful habits, can supplement pharmaceutical interventions and promote longevity.

Medication Adherence: Patients should be educated on the importance of medication adherence, which includes taking medications as prescribed and not stopping them without consulting with a healthcare provider.

Research and Development: In the pharmaceutical industry, ongoing research and development is critical to discovering safer and more effective medications, as well as innovative therapies that can further extend longevity.

Pharmaceutical drugs have unquestionably increased life expectancy and quality of life. However, they should always be used under the supervision of a healthcare professional, with the goal of optimizing health while minimizing risks.

To live a longer and healthier life, an integrated approach that combines pharmaceutical interventions with healthy lifestyle choices is essential.

Practice Preventative Healthcare: Regular check-ups, health screenings, and vaccinations can help prevent chronic diseases and detect health issues early on. Regular preventative healthcare can also help manage chronic conditions and reduce the risk of complications.

Longevity and its Risks

Longevity, the gift of extended life, has long been a cherished aspiration of humanity.

It represents the triumph of science, medicine, and social progress over the relentless grasp of mortality. However, beneath the surface of this remarkable achievement lies a multitude of challenges that require careful consideration and thoughtful navigation.

First and foremost, the challenge of longevity lies in ensuring that these added years are not just measured in quantity but also in quality.

Prolonged life should be marked by vitality, purpose, and fulfilment rather than a mere extension of frailty and suffering.

This means addressing the burden of chronic diseases, cognitive decline, and physical debilitation that often accompany ageing.

It demands innovative approaches to healthcare, emphasizing prevention and early intervention, as well as the development of technologies and therapies that enhance the human body's resilience against the ravages of time.

Moreover, as we extend our lifespans, we must confront the economic implications of a growing elderly population.

Traditional pension systems and healthcare infrastructures were not designed to accommodate such demographic shifts.

Adequate financial planning, sustainable retirement strategies, and adaptable social support systems become imperative to ensure that longevity is not a recipe for economic hardship and intergenerational inequalities.

The psychological and social dimensions of longevity also present profound challenges.

People living longer may experience a sense of displacement, as the roles and expectations associated with different stages of life evolve. Relationships, too, may be tested, as families grapple with the dynamics of caring for aging parents or partners.

Loneliness and social isolation can become increasingly prevalent, necessitating a reimagining of community structures and support networks to foster meaningful connections and combat the silent epidemic of solitude.

The environmental impact of a longer-lived population cannot be overlooked. Longer lifespans mean greater resource consumption and potential strains on ecosystems.

Sustainability becomes a crucial consideration, necessitating responsible consumption patterns, innovative energy solutions, and environmentally friendly technologies to mitigate our impact on the planet.

In our pursuit of longevity, we must also navigate the ethical dilemmas that arise.

Questions surrounding the equitable distribution of life-extending technologies, access to healthcare, and the potential for social disparities to widen must be addressed with sensitivity and fairness.

Balancing individual desires for extended life with the broader societal interest in resource allocation is a delicate ethical tightrope.

While the prospect of longevity is a testament to human progress and ingenuity, it carries with it an array of complex challenges.

Addressing these challenges requires a multifaceted approach, involving advances in healthcare, economics, psychology, sociology, and ethics.

It calls for a collective commitment to ensure that the gift of a longer life is not overshadowed by the burdens it may bring.

Only by tackling these challenges with wisdom and compassion can we truly harness the potential of longevity to enrich our lives and the world we inhabit.

Conclusion

We've embarked on a trip through the enthralling landscape of longevity, investigating scientific as well as cultural insights, and personal experiences that throw light on the age-old search for a longer and more satisfying life.

As we conclude this investigation, it's worth pausing to consider the varied character of longevity and its significant consequences for humans.

Longevity, we've realized, is a holistic and diverse quest, not just a matter of prolonging the years we spend in this world.

It includes not only technological advances and medical breakthroughs that allow us to withstand the ravages of time, but also the social, psychological, and spiritual aspects of our existence.

We've discussed the significance of living a healthy lifestyle, including adequate eating, frequent exercise, and mindfulness techniques.

We've learnt that our genes influence our longevity, but they don't have the last say. Our decisions, behaviours, and surroundings all have a big impact on how we age.

We've also looked at the role of our connections and relationships in living a long and fulfilling life.

Loneliness and social isolation have emerged as invisible risks to our well-being, emphasizing the significance of creating community and obtaining emotional assistance.

The wisdom of centenarians, those exceptional individuals who have not only conquered the odds but have done so with elegance, tenacity, and purpose, has also graced the pages of this book.

Their experiences remind us that longevity is about the quality of those years, not the quantity of years. It is about discovering purpose, following one's passions, and leaving a lasting legacy.

The goal of longevity is a very personal and communal endeavour. It challenges us to reflect on our beliefs, priorities, and the legacy we want to leave for future generations.

It encourages us to take a more holistic approach to health and well-being, one that considers not only the physical aspects of aging but also the emotional, social, and existential factors.

Let us carry forward the knowledge, insights, and inspiration gained from these pages as we close this chapter.

Let us go on our own individual paths to a longer, better, and more meaningful life. And let us do it with the understanding that the search of longevity is a profound examination of what it is to be human, not just a scientific or medical undertaking.

www.ingramcontent.com/pod-product-compliance
Lightning Source LLC
Chambersburg PA
CBHW070721260726
48660CB00007B/2668